1085

Foreword

The College set up a Working Party under the Chairmanship of Professor A in November 1996 in response to questions raised in parliament relating to fetal pain and awareness, and subsequent articles in the media. The College felt that it was important to review the available evidence in relation to this subject.

The Working Party has reviewed in great depth all available published material, examined current practice in relation to intrauterine procedures carried out during pregnancy and considered the need for change in future practice.

I hope it will be possible to obtain the necessary funding to undertake the research outlined in their report.

I would like to thank Professor McLaren and her Working Party for all the hardwork, time and effort they have given to the preparation of this important Report; which is extremely well written and very informative.

I would also like to thank the Department of Health for their support.

Naren Patel
President

McLean A

Further copies of this report can be obtained from:

The RCOG Bookshop
The Royal College of Obstetricians and Gynaecologists
27 Sussex Place
Regent's Park
London
NW1 4RG

Tel. No: (0171) 772 6275/276
Fax. No: (0171) 724 5991
email: bookshop@rcog.org.uk
website: www.rcog.org.uk

Registered Charity No: 213280

ISBN 1 900364 07 7

Published by the RCOG Press

CONTENTS

Membership

Professor Anne McLaren, DBE, FRS, FRCOG - Chairman
Wellcome/CRC Institute, Cambridge

Professor Albert Aynsley-Green, FRCP, FRCP (Edin) FRCPCH, Institute of Child Health, University College London Medical School

Professor Margaret Brazier, LLB, Barrister, Institute of Medicine, Law and Bioethics, University of Manchester

Professor The Reverend Canon Gordon R Dunstan, CBE, DD, LLD, FRCOG

Professor Maria Fitzgerald, BA, PhD, Department of Anatomy and Developmental Biology, University College London

Dr Ian A F Lister-Cheese, FRCP, FRCPCH, Medical Adviser, Department of Health (Observer)

Professor Neil McIntosh, FRCP, FRCPCH, Department of Child Life and Health, University of Edinburgh

Professor Kypros Nicolaides, MRCOG, Harris Birthright Research Centre for Fetal Medicine

Professor Felicity Reynolds, MD, FRCA, FRCOG, Emeritus Professor of Obstetric Anaesthesia, St Thomas' Hospital, London

Professor Stephen Robson, MD, MRCOG, Department of Fetal Medicine, University of Newcastle upon Tyne

Professor Charles Rodeck, DSc(Med), FRCOG, FRCPath, Department of Obstetrics and Gynaecology, University College London Medical School

ACKNOWLEDGEMENTS

The Working Party would like to thank the following:-

Professor Peter Hepper, Director, Wellcome Trust Fetal Behaviour Research Centre, Queen's University of Belfast, who provided a written submission to the Working Party.

All the clinics that responded to the survey on anaesthesia during termination of pregnancy referred to in section 3.6.

Terms of Reference

- To review evidence relating to fetal awareness.

- To document current practice in relation to intrauterine procedures during pregnancy.

- To consider the need for change in practice and make appropriate recommendations.

* **Note: the gestational age used throughout this report is measured from last menstrual period (LMP)**

1.   Summary and Recommendations

1.1   Summary

Concerns generated by debate on fetal awareness caused the Royal College of Obstetricians and Gynaecologists to establish a Working Party to examine the subject in detail. The Working Party included experts in fetal and neonatal medicine, anaesthesia, biological and neurological scientists and two lay people, a theologian and a lawyer.

The Working Party's underlying principle was that the fetus should be protected from any potentially painful or harmful procedures but that the assessment of whether the fetus might conceivably be able to feel pain or might be harmed in either the short or long term must be based on established scientific evidence.

The Working Party took the view that their Report should be written so that it stood up to scientific scrutiny but was also understandable to a wide audience.

In considering the difficult issue of fetal awareness and termination of pregnancy, the Working Party wishes to emphasise that the ethics of late terminations must be kept separate from the ethical issues raised by the possibility of fetal pain.

The main findings and conclusions of the Working Party were as follows:

- Awareness depends upon the structural and functional integration of the cerebral cortex with other parts of the central nervous system and the peripheral nervous system.

- It is possible by direct means to identify the minimum stage of structural development that is **necessary_-** but not that which is sufficient - to confer awareness upon the developing fetus. This minimum stage of development, with structural integration of peripheral nerves, spinal cord, brain stem, thalamus and, finally, the cerebral cortex, **has not begun before 26 weeks' gestation**.

- Structural and functional development of the nervous system continues until adult life. During this time the point is reached when it may be said that awareness is possible. That point cannot be identified precisely but the quality of awareness becomes evident during infancy.

- Before the state of development necessary for awareness is reached, other events occur which are mediated by the fetal nervous system. Among them are:-

    (i) From 5-6 weeks' gestation the neuromuscular system is sufficiently developed for spontaneous fetal movements to occur. This happens before peripheral sensory nerves are linked to the central nervous system.

(ii) Sensory nerves first grow into the spinal cord at 14 weeks' gestation. It is probable that these nerves transmit impulses arising from non-noxious stimuli, such as touch.

(iii) Nerves that transmit impulses arising from noxious stimuli have not made connection with the spinal cord by 19 weeks' gestation.

(iv) The pre-term infant of 23 weeks' gestation shows reflex responses to noxious stimuli.

- Other events that are mediated through the peripheral and central nervous systems are the physiological, hormonal and metabolic responses to noxious stimuli. They are called stress responses, a term used to describe the responses of an organism to stimuli which signify a threat.

- Stress responses are not always commensurate with the threat. The term does not imply suffering, pain or awareness of these happenings although it does not preclude them.

- Contrary to popular belief there is no major "surgery" on the fetus being performed in the United Kingdom. A number of diagnostic tests are carried out on fetuses but most of these do not involve any direct contact with the fetus. Fetal analgesia is not routinely given for the majority of such procedures.

- However, in those few procedures that involve direct contact with the fetus, such as inserting a needle or catheter into the fetus itself, the possibility of pain in the later stages of pregnancy (after 24` weeks' gestation) must be considered.

- Agents given to the mother to provide general anaesthesia or sedation will cross the placenta and affect the fetus but this occurs more slowly than in the mother.

- Stress responses in the fetus and newborn can be attenuated by analgesic and anaesthetic agents. It is widely accepted that infants who undergo procedures which generate sustained stress responses, and which in older children would be painful, should receive these agents. This view has been promoted, at least in part, by the duty to relieve or prevent pain, even when its occurrence is uncertain. We conclude that similar consideration should be given to the fetus beyond 24 weeks' gestation. However, it is not known whether the use of these agents alters subsequent development and normal physiological or behavioural responsiveness. This is an important area for study.

1.2 Recommendations

1. We **recommend** that practitioners who undertake diagnostic or therapeutic surgical procedures upon the fetus at or after 24 weeks' gestation (which takes account of the uncertainty that attends estimates of gestational age) consider the requirements for fetal analgesia and sedation.

2. We **recommend** that practitioners who undertake termination of pregnancy at 24 weeks or later should consider the requirements for feticide or fetal analgesia and sedation.

3. We **recommend** that further research be undertaken into the subjects identified at 5.2.

2.   Introduction

2 .1   The Problem

The Working Party was asked to review the evidence relating to fetal awareness. We first considered the evidence on responses to sensory stimuli, including both early reflex responses to light or sound, and fetal "memory" of, for example, the theme tunes of television programmes watched by the mother during pregnancy.[1] All of these could be conditioned reflexes. We decided that in the present context it was awareness of pain that the College and the public were interested in, and accordingly concentrated on that.

The Working Party addressed four questions:
- Might a fetus be aware of pain?
- If so, at what stage might this ability develop?
- Is it in the future interests of a surviving baby to attempt to alleviate any such sensations?
- What are the implications for the practice of obstetrics and gynaecology in relation both to diagnostic and therapeutic procedures carried out on the fetus and to the termination of pregnancy, when the fetus is not expected to survive?

2.2   What is Awareness?

The Working Party made no attempt to define awareness, pain, consciousness or sentience. Definitions tend to be circular and philosophers have written whole books on consciousness. "Awareness" and "pain" are both multi-layered phenomena incorporating cognitive as well as physiological elements. In the fetus it is impossible to ascertain the relationship between these two elements. We are, however, agreed that a simple physical reaction to stimuli is not by itself evidence of cognitive awareness or pain.

Research has shown that the neurological connections enabling reflex reaction to stimulation develop some time before the fetal brain is sufficiently advanced to allow any possibility of awareness. The Working Party considered the evidence as to the nature of awareness and concluded that they accepted the consensus of neuroscientific opinion that awareness is a cortical phenomenon.[2] It follows that fetal awareness of pain is impossible until at least the time that sensory connections first penetrate the cortex. Furthermore, whereas the arrival of this sensory information is **necessary**, we do not consider that it is **sufficient** for the perception of pain, which will require the growth of interconnections between many brain areas and the maturation of the transmission of electrical and chemical messages, all of which are slow processes stretching well into infancy. It is important therefore to consider the possible long term consequences of noxious stimulation or tissue damage to the immature nervous system of surviving fetuses as well as the long term effects of the administration of powerful analgesics at a time of rapid neural development.[3] Animal research has shown that even stimuli of which a fetus is unaware may permanently alter the future development of the nervous system.[4] In newborn infants, relatively minor surgery, such as circumcision, has been shown to alter pain reactions several months later.[5]

These factors need to be considered when undertaking intrauterine diagnostic and therapeutic procedures involving contact with the fetus and procedures for late termination of pregnancy. The purpose of this report is to examine current practice and to consider whether, in the light of current knowledge, changes are required.

3.   Current Practice

3.1   Invasive Diagnostic Procedures

Women whose fetuses are at increased risk of chromosomal or genetic diseases may choose to have diagnostic procedures. The great majority of these do not involve any fetal contact.

3.1.1   *Diagnostic procedures not involving fetal contact*

These include:-

- Amniocentesis;

- Chorion villus sampling (or placental biopsy);

- Fetal blood sampling from the umbilical cord (cordocentesis);

- Embryoscopy or fetoscopy.

These are all performed with careful ultrasound guidance so that the fetus is not touched or damaged. The placenta and umbilical cord have no nerve supply and are not capable of either receiving or transmitting sensation.

Amniocentesis is by far the most common (some 30,000 in the UK per annum). A fine needle (less than 1mm in diameter) is passed through the mother's abdominal wall and into the amniotic cavity, within which the fetus lies, usually at 15 to 16 weeks' gestation. About 10-20 ml of amniotic fluid are withdrawn.

Chorion villus sampling is less common (about 3,000 per annum in the UK). It can be performed either through the mother's abdomen, like amniocentesis, or through the cervix. It is mostly carried out at 10 to 14 weeks' gestation.

Fetal blood sampling is becoming uncommon (less than 1,000 per annum in the UK) as it is increasingly possible to obtain the same information using simpler tests such as amniocentesis or chorion villus sampling. The most accessible point for sampling is usually the attachment of the umbilical cord to the placenta, into which a fine needle is passed, with ultrasound guidance.

Embryoscopy or fetoscopy enables the direct inspection of fetal anatomy by passing a fine endoscope (up to 2 mm diameter) through the abdominal wall. These procedures are seldom used because ultrasound, which is non-invasive, nearly always provides sufficiently accurate information.

3.1.2   *Diagnostic procedures involving fetal contact or puncture*

These are:-

- Fetal blood sampling from the umbilical vein in the fetal liver (about 200 are performed per annum in the UK).

- Withdrawal of fluid from a cyst or cystic organ such as the bladder (about 75 procedures are performed per annum in the UK).

- Biopsy of fetal skin, liver, muscle, tumour or other tissue (less than 20 per annum in the UK).

Fetal analgesia or **sedation** are not normally given.

3.2   Invasive Therapeutic Procedures

The two main approaches are "open" surgery , in which an incision is made in the mother's abdomen and then through the wall of the uterus, and percutaneous procedures in which a needle or fine tube is inserted through the mother's skin and into the uterus.

3.2.1   *"Open" surgery*

This involves a major operation on the mother allowing surgery directly on the fetus.[6] No such highly invasive surgery is currently carried out in the UK; at present it is confined **to two or three centres mainly in the USA**.

3.2.2   *Percutaneous procedures*

These procedures are carried out with ultrasound guidance under local anaesthesia to the mother. The great majority do not involve any direct fetal contact and are usually carried out between 20 and 34 weeks' gestation.

Percutaneous Procedures without fetal contact

These include:-

- Transfusion of blood or platelets into the umbilical cord if the fetus is anaemic or deficient in platelets.

- Fetoscopic laser ablation of vessels on the placental surface in the twin-twin transfusion syndrome.

- Fetoscopic ligation of the umbilical cord, for the same indication.

The first of these is the most common and most successful form of fetal therapy. The other two are still under evaluation. None involves the fetus or areas capable of sensation.

---

[*] This figure is derived from the survey referred to in section 3.4. The survey did not seek to distinguish between diagnostic and therapeutic access to the intra-hepatic umbilical vein and the figure given is therefore an estimate of the number of *diagnostic* procedures. This caveat also applies to the number given for *therapeutic* procedures involving access to the intra-hepatic umbilical vein in section 3.2.2. above.

Percutaneous therapeutic procedures that involve direct fetal contact

These are of three main types:-

- Transfusion into the intra-hepatic umbilical vein of the fetus, the heart, or the peritoneal cavity - about 100 are performed per annum in the UK (see footnote on page (8)).

- Drainage of abnormal fluid collections, for example in the bladder or the chest, by introducing a shunt (a plastic catheter, 2 mm in diameter). About 50 are performed per annum in the UK.

- A number of endoscopic procedures are being evaluated. At present, very few have been performed.

Some of these procedures are carried out with maternal sedation as well as local anaesthesia. The fetus may then be sedated and immobile. However, this may be disadvantageous since the success of the procedure may depend on fetal mobility and fetal movements may assist, for example, in the expulsion of fluids through a shunt.

3.3 Selective Termination and Multifetal Pregnancy Reduction

Feticide, bringing about the death of one or more fetuses, may be used in a continuing multiple pregnancy if one or more of the fetuses is severely abnormal or if the number of fetuses is too great for the health of the mother or the maintenance of the pregnancy.

The most widely used method is an injection of potassium chloride into the fetal chest cavity or heart (depending on the size of the fetus) which ensures instant cessation of the heart beat. Fetal anaesthesia is not usually given. Techniques avoiding fetal contact include stopping the fetal heart by coagulation of the cord vessels using an ultrasonically directed probe.

Multi-fetal pregnancy reduction is usually performed in the late first or early second trimester, before 14 weeks, by injection of potassium chloride into the chest cavity.

3.4 Administration of Analgesics during Intrauterine Procedures

To document current practice, a questionnaire was sent to fetal medicine specialists in the nine largest units in the UK. These fetal medicine units are likely to be performing the greatest number of intrauterine procedures involving fetal contact. Replies were received from all nine and were presented to the College's Scientific Advisory Committee in 1996.

Of the eight units undertaking fetal blood sampling from the hepatic vein (median number of samplings per year =25 [range 3-70]), two had a policy of administering parenteral analgesia to the mother before the procedure. Fetal shunting (chest or bladder) was undertaken in all nine units (median number of shunts per year =6 [range 2-25]). Five respondents stated that parenteral analgesia was given to the mother before the procedure. All units performed other procedures involving fetal contact (e.g. urine sampling, skin biopsy) and four had a policy of administering analgesia to the mother. Where analgesia was given this was always in the form of an intramuscular opioid (omnopon 10-15 mg, pethidine 20-50 mg or diamorphine 5-10 mg) administered within one hour of the procedure.

In no unit was analgesia routinely administered directly to the fetus for any of these procedures although one respondent gave fentanyl 3-10 µg per kg estimated fetal weight as part of a research protocol. One other respondent commented that in cases of late selective feticide, the fetus was given diazemuls and ketamine. The attention of the Working Party was drawn to the fact that at least two other centres are carrying out research projects in this area.

3.5 Termination of Pregnancy

The methods for termination of pregnancy can be classified into surgical and medical (Table 1). Surgical terminations are usually carried out under general anaesthesia, especially at gestations beyond 10 weeks. Medical terminations are usually carried out under maternal sedation and analgesia, especially after 12 weeks. Terminations after 24 weeks are only permitted for serious fetal abnormalities.

3.5.1 *Surgical termination*

(a) Cervical dilatation and removal of the fetus
For pregnancies beyond 10 weeks, surgical dilatation of the cervix is usually preceded by medical preparation of the cervix. Before 12-14 weeks the fetus, placenta and membranes (products of conception) are removed by suction through a cannula and fetal death is instantaneous. After 14 weeks, there is piecemeal removal of the uterine contents and death of the fetus occurs within a few seconds.

(b) Hysterotomy (incision of the uterus)
This is carried out for fetuses with abnormalities where vaginal delivery is impossible either because of placenta praevia or pelvic tumour, or because of fetal abnormality such as conjoined twins. It is also occasionally carried out in cases of failed medical termination.

(c) Hysterectomy (removal of the uterus)
This is carried out only for serious maternal conditions, usually malignancy, and is confined to gestations below 24 weeks. Hysterectomy for maternal indications at viable gestations is preceded by caesarean delivery.

FIGURE 1

FETAL INTERVENTION

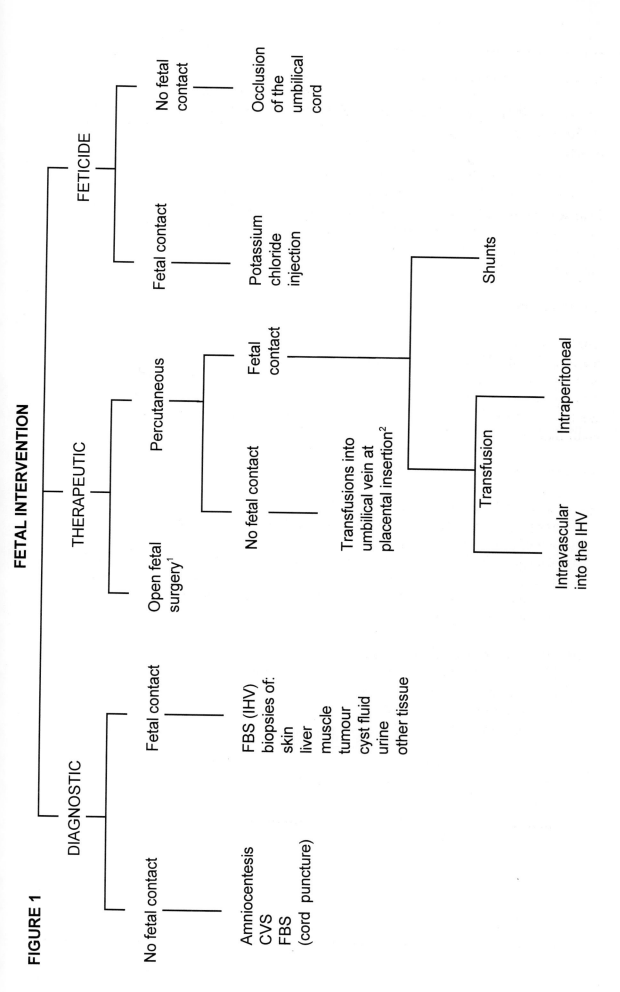

1. Not currently performed in the UK.
2. By far the commonest of the therapeutic procedures.

CVS = chorion villus sampling; FBS = fetal blood sampling; IHV = intrahepatic vein

Table 1

ENGLAND & WALES RESIDENTS: LEGAL TERMINATIONS OF PREGNANCIES 1995 BY METHOD AND PERIOD OF GESTATION.

Source: Office for National Statistics, Abortion Statistics Series AB No. 22. (Additional information on abortions by method over 25 weeks' gestation supplied by direct correspondence with the ONS)

Gestation (weeks)	0-12	13-19	20-24	25 and over	Total
Surgical (abdominal)	34	14	16	2	66
Surgical (vaginal)	130,879	11,489	675	0	143,043
Surgical (not specified)	0	2	2	1	5
Medical	6,757	3,233	1,072	57	11,119
Combined methods	26	47	7	2	82
Total (all methods)	**137,696**	**14,785**	**1,772**	**62**	**154,315**

Table 2

ENGLAND & WALES RESIDENTS; NUMBER OF TERMINATIONS PERFORMED BEYOND 24 WEEKS' GESTATION; 1995

(Source: Office for National Statistics, Abortion Statistics Series AB No. 22.)

Gestational Age in Weeks	Number of Terminations
25-28	36
29-33	20
34-38	6
Total	**62**

(Note: Table 1 includes the numbers in Table 2)

Prostaglandins, with or without anti-progesterone agents, may be given to women having medical terminations after 14 weeks. These produce uterine contractions and cervical dilatation causing a miscarriage, usually within 24 hours. If there are retained products the procedure is completed by surgical evacuation under general anaesthesia.

When a pregnancy is terminated because of fetal abnormality after 21 weeks, the procedure, either surgical or medical, is usually preceded by injection of potassium chloride into the umbilical cord or fetal heart in order to stop the fetal heart beat.[7]

An alternative method of stopping the fetal heart before termination of pregnancy is to cut the umbilical cord after dilatation of the cervix and immediately before the onset of surgical evacuation of the fetus and placenta. This procedure is carried out under general anaesthesia.

3.6   Anaesthesia During Termination of Pregnancy

In modern anaesthetic practice it has become customary to avoid heavy premedication particularly in outpatients and for short procedures so that hangover is minimised. In such circumstances the patient is rapidly anaesthetised but doses of all drugs are kept to a minimum, so that the patient wakes quickly and the danger of semi-consciousness during the postoperative period is reduced.

Anaesthetists working in all clinics approved to perform terminations at 20-24 weeks' gestation were asked to provide information on whether premedication was used, what agents and doses were used for induction and maintenance of anaesthesia, and how soon after induction of anaesthesia the procedure was started.

- All replied that no sedative premedication was given (in one case antacid prophylaxis was given as premedication; this has no sedative properties).
- All used propofol, in doses between 175 and 250 mg or methohexitone 150-175 mg, with fentanyl or alfentanil for induction of anaesthesia. Half of the respondents also added a benzodiazepine, either diazepam or midazolam. One third added an antiemetic, either droperidol or metoclopramide.
- For maintenance of anaesthesia all gave nitrous oxide, with either increments of propofol or a volatile agent, either enflurane or isoflurane.
- All stated that the procedure was started either immediately after induction of anaesthesia or within 2-3 minutes.

In NHS units where medical termination is undertaken after the twentieth week of pregnancy, either epidural analgesia or large doses of diamorphine may be given to the mother. Epidural analgesia is desirable for the sake of the mother both because pain relief is superior and because it may be necessary to evacuate retained products of conception. In the absence of epidural blockade this would necessitate general anaesthesia which carries greater risk.

4. Summary of Current Knowledge of Fetal Awareness

4.1   The Development of Sensory Pathways in the Human Fetus (Figure 2)

The awareness of sensory stimulation on or within the body is not necessarily sufficient to allow the feeling of pain. Cognitive activities, such as memories of past experiences, attention and suggestion, all contribute to pain experience.[8] Indeed in some adult pathological states it is possible to feel pain in the absence of an obvious stimulus. However, in relation to the fetus, we consider that the formation of sensory connections linking the skin and underlying organs of the body through peripheral nerves to the spinal cord and brainstem, and from there to the thalamus and up to the cerebral cortex, is a prerequisite to any possibility of sensory experience and pain. These data have been thoroughly reviewed elsewhere.[9-13] Much of our knowledge arises from the study of laboratory animals but relevant data on human development will be briefly summarised below.

4.1.1   *Sensory innervation of the skin*

Sensory innervation of the fetal skin has been reported to begin very early in the first trimester[14] although it should be noted that it is largely subdermal (below the surface layers) at this stage. After 28 weeks' gestation nerve endings are also seen near the surface.[15]

4.1.2   *Sensory connections in the spinal cord*

In order to carry information to the central nervous system, these sensory nerves need to grow into the spinal cord, via the dorsal roots, and to make connections with neurons in the dorsal part of the spinal cord. In the human fetus the first sensory fibres grow into the spinal cord at 14 weeks' gestation and animal studies show that these fibres are likely to transmit touch and other non-noxious information. Noxious information is carried by small diameter fibres (called C fibres) which terminate in the superficial parts of the spinal dorsal horn and at 19 weeks' gestation these have still not formed connections in the spinal cord.[16]

4.1.3   *Reflex movements*

Spontaneous fetal movements can be detected by real-time ultrasound from 7.5-8 weeks' gestation.[17] Reflex responses to touching the region of the mouth are also reported to begin at this time but these reflex data should be treated with caution since they were obtained from exteriorised fetuses during termination.[18] Such fetuses would be severely deprived of oxygen and this can result in general muscle twitching. The time of onset of responses to noxious stimulation is unknown but, as discussed above in section 4.1.2, these are unlikely to be before 19 weeks' gestation.[16] Reflex responses to noxious stimuli can be evoked in the youngest preterm infant (23 weeks' gestational age) but their properties are different from those of the adult in a number of ways.[19] They are larger in amplitude, of longer duration, can also be evoked by low intensity, non-noxious stimulation and can be activated from a larger area of the body surface than adult reflexes. This has led to the conclusion that there are considerable differences in the reflex connections between the immature and the adult spinal cord.

4.1.4 *The Thalamus*

The thalamus is the major subcortical nucleus through which all painful stimuli are transmitted en route to the cortex. Several thalamic nuclei are involved in processing normal pain sensation in animals and humans.[20] It has been argued that thalamic activity alone may be capable of generating a 'dull' sensation of pain or discomfort. There is no evidence for this proposition but it has been raised in relation to the issue of fetal awareness since cortical connections develop relatively late in fetal life but thalamic function may mature earlier.

At 6 weeks the thalamus is a poorly differentiated structure on the sides of the third ventricle. From 6-8 weeks' gestation differentiation begins and the ventricular zone, intermediate zone and mantle zone can be distinguished along with some bipolar radially arranged neurons. From 10-14 weeks' gestation segregation of neurons into groups or nuclei begins and some neurons have grown primary dendrites. From 14-16 weeks' gestation segregation continues, neurons are maturing and some multipolar neurons with longer branched dendrites appear.[21] Myelination first occurs in the thalamus along with other subcortical structures, globus pallidus and posterior internal capsule at 25 weeks' gestation, well before the cortex at 35 weeks' gestation.[22] In one of the major thalamic nuclei (the lateral geniculate nucleus involved in visual processing), which has been well studied, synaptic contacts (connections for transmission between neurons) are not observed until 13-14 weeks' gestation. These arise from the retina but are notably immature at this age. The period from 15-20 weeks' gestation is marked by a great increase in both the number and the maturation of these synapses but they do not begin to acquire the pattern and structure seen in the adult until 20-21 weeks' gestation.[23] It should be noted that only 40% of the synaptic input of the thalamus is from sensory pathways arising from the spinal cord, brainstem or retina; the remaining 60% is from the cortex, in the form of descending connections. These do not reach the thalamus before 20-21 weeks' gestation.[23] This is important because thalamic function beyond a simple relay or filter system is dependent on feedback from the cortex.[24] These descending fibres only transmit nerve impulses from cortex to thalamus, not in the reverse direction.

In conclusion, the thalamus begins to mature earlier than the cortex but its function beyond a simple relay depends on connections with higher levels of the nervous system which do not begin before 22 weeks' gestation.

4.1.5   *The Cortex*

A functional cortex is essential if the fetus is to be aware or to perceive external events. Reports from brain damaged or abnormal adults claiming to show that pain or other sensations can be felt in the absence of a functional cortex are not relevant here as they are referring to a mature and fully connected, albeit dysfunctional, nervous system. In fetal life, if the cortex is to be functional, it requires sensory input from the thalamus. Furthermore, it requires intrinsic circuitry and connections with other brain areas to be established. Relatively little is known about human cortical development but a critical fact is that thalamocortical connections are first observed penetrating the frontal cortical plate at 26-34 weeks' gestation.[25] Therefore, before that time there is no sensory input to the cortex. Widespread and diffuse monoamine-containing axons start to grow into the primitive cortex from as early as 16 weeks[25a] but these do not carry sensory information. They are likely to be involved in the growth and guidance of neural connections in the immature cortex. Evoked potential studies support this, showing that the distinct component signalling the arrival of sensory impulses at a cortical level can be detected at 29 weeks' gestation.[26] However, to suggest that the arrival of sensory signals in these first fibres is in itself sufficient to allow awareness of pain is contrary to our understanding of central nervous function. Maturation of the human cortex is a prolonged process and depends upon the sensory input acquired in late fetal and postnatal life. New neurons are still being generated at 34 weeks' gestation and synaptogenesis continues for two years, stimulated and modified in the light of sensory experience. Recent imaging studies emphasise that there is no single cortical area associated with a sensation of pain, but rather many different cortical areas are activated when painful stimuli are perceived.[27] Structural and functional development of the nervous system continues until adult life. During this time the point is reached when it may be said that awareness is possible. That point cannot be identified precisely but the quality of awareness becomes evident during infancy.

FIGURE 2

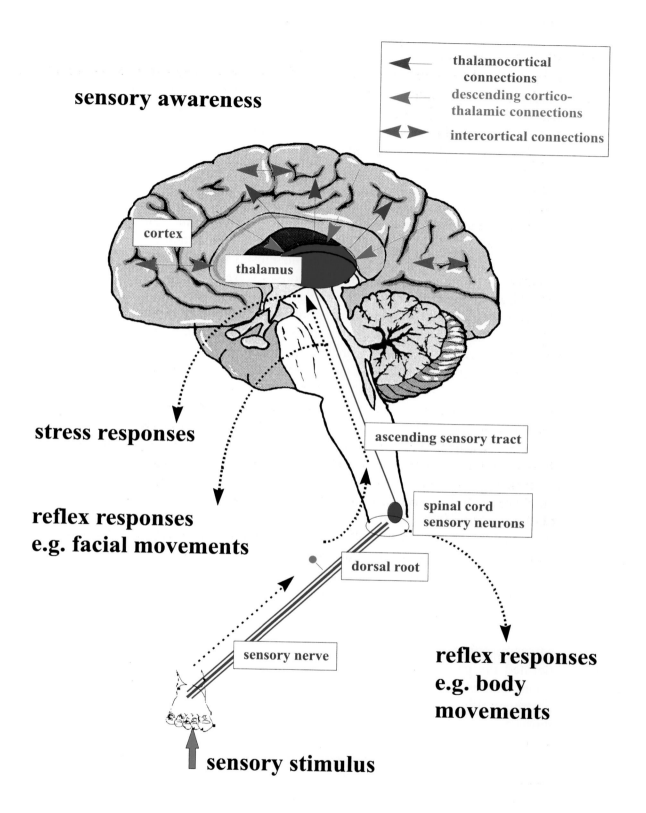

A schematic diagram of sensory pathways in the brain, showing the levels of reflex and stress responses and the thalamic and cortical connections involved in awareness.

4.2 Fetal Responsiveness to Adverse Stimuli

Study of the responses of the fetal nervous system to adverse or noxious stimuli is necessarily indirect. Reflex movements, while useful, are confounded by the presence of on-going spontaneous fetal movements and by the fact that they can also be evoked by non-noxious stimuli. Changes in heart rate are equally unreliable. The measurement of certain hormones and metabolites in fetal blood has been used as a more selective, chemical indicator of the responses mounted by the fetal nervous system to noxious stimuli. They are called stress responses.

In the 1980s it was established that newborn babies were able to mount a stress response to acute surgery implying that they were feeling pain.[28,29] These stress responses were, however, different from those observed in adults both in duration and magnitude. Research into the use of analgesics when performing operations on newborn babies showed that stress responses were diminished and postoperative complications were reduced when analgesics and anaesthetics were used.[30,31] This led to a consensus that newborn babies were able to feel pain and raised the possibility that the unborn fetus was also capable of feeling pain at some stage of its development. Recent work on fetuses undergoing intrauterine procedures has shown that they are indeed able to mount similar stress responses.[32]

Stress in lay parlance is conscious and emotional and thought to be detrimental to well-being. Stress, however, is used in a particular way in medicine. Biologically, the stress response is necessary for survival, either as the "fight or flight" phenomenon or as the hormonal and metabolic response to tissue damage that initiates repair. There is evidence that in the fetus and infant such responses have a part in normal development. The term does not imply suffering, pain or awareness of these happenings, although it does not preclude them. Stress responses can occur in the unconscious or anaesthetised subject. For example in adult subjects undergoing removal of the gall bladder it is possible to abolish pain by a combination of epidural and general anaesthesia but the stress responses remain pronounced.[33] Thus, awareness is not a pre-requisite for the generation of stress responses in the adult.

Stress responses are not always commensurate with the threat. Recent work has defined the patterns of metabolic and endocrine responses to medical illness in young babies. Such infants aged 3-6 months suffering from acute bronchiolitis and gastroenteritis demonstrate plasma stress hormone levels which are similar to those seen at the end of major surgery.[34] In these circumstances it would be harmful to administer powerful analgesics to decrease the stress responses. Furthermore, substantial stress responses are seen in older children with major head injury despite the fact that they are unconscious.[35] Finally, stress responses still occur in healthy older children subjected to elective surgery under current state-of-the-art anaesthesia.[36] Since, as in the adult, stress can be demonstrated in children in circumstances in which consciousness and awareness are not present, it has been argued that it is too simplistic to suggest that a stress response is synonymous with the experience of pain in children.[32,37]

Stress responses have evolved because of their survival value in post-natal life. The fetus, however, is protected from most noxious or harmful stimuli. Although stress responses in mature form do not exist in the fetus, immature versions of these responses can be seen in late gestation. As with other activities, they develop *in utero* in readiness for extrauterine life.

What then is the function of these responses in the fetus? Are they useful or harmful? Probably in both fetus and neonate, an acute short term response to pain or stress could be beneficial, whereas a chronic response may be more harmful.

By way of example the process of birth is an acute stimulus and although there is no evidence that it is painful for the fetus (unlike the mother), it causes a stress response which is a vital part of the adaptation to extrauterine life. For example the release of catecholamines promotes the absorption of lung fluid at birth. Babies that have experienced labour, however delivered (whether vaginally or by caesarean), adapt better than those delivered by elective caesarean *without* labour.

Stress responses in the fetus and the newborn can be attenuated by analgesic and anaesthetic agents. It is widely accepted that infants who undergo procedures which generate sustained stress responses which in older children would be painful should receive these agents. This view has been promoted largely by the duty to relieve or prevent pain, even when its occurrence is uncertain. However, it is not known whether the use of such agents at this stage of development affects subsequent physiological or behavioural development, including normal responsiveness to adverse influences. This is an important area for study.

Even some chronic stresses may confer advantages: the fetus that is small-for-gestational age due to nutritional deprivation may behave in a more mature manner after birth than a normally grown fetus of the same gestational age. For example it may breathe better. It is thought that prolonged intrauterine stress may increase the production of steroids which promote the maturation of a number of organs such as the lungs.

4. 3   The Effects of Analgesic and Anaesthetic Drugs on the Fetus

Obstetric anaesthetists are usually concerned that, for any drug they may give to the mother when the baby is about to be born, the effect on the baby should be minimal. It is generally considered desirable that any analgesia and anaesthesia given shortly before birth should not impair the ability of the newborn to adapt to extrauterine life. This is not a concern in termination of pregnancy.

Concern about the possible need for fetal analgesia during intrauterine procedures or late terminations raises the opposite problem. In these circumstances, if fetal awareness is considered a possibility, and if, in the case of late termination, feticide is not practised, it becomes important to consider how best to achieve effective fetal sedation or analgesia.

Our understanding of the effects on the baby of maternal analgesia and anaesthesia stems principally from studies following either caesarean section under general anaesthesia or the use of systemic drugs for pain relief and, in the past, sedation during labour.

4.3.1 *Placental transfer of drugs*

The surface of the placenta is covered with a continuous lipid membrane, so lipid-insoluble substances, such as those needed for growth and metabolism, require specialised transport processes to enable them to traverse it. Foreign substances such as drugs can only cross the placenta readily by lipid diffusion, following normal physical laws. The result is that lipid-soluble drugs come into equilibrium across the placenta rapidly (in the non-ionised and unbound form), but water-soluble drugs cross only slowly, and indeed do not come into transplacental equilibrium.[38]

Drugs acting on the central nervous system to produce unconsciousness or even analgesia must all cross the blood-brain (or blood-spinal cord) barrier and therefore must be lipid-soluble. Inevitably, therefore, they cross the placenta with as much ease as the blood-brain barrier. Nevertheless, the fetus is what is termed a deep compartment, and though many such drugs come into equilibrium across the placenta in a single placental circulation, full equilibration with the entire fetal compartment is delayed.[38] This is easily understood if one takes into account the obvious fact that maternal blood does not circulate through fetal tissues but only through the maternal side of the placenta.

4.3.2 *General anaesthesia*

It is well recognised that a baby born by caesarean section without undue delay is fully alert, whereas if there is delay and difficulty in delivering the baby, it becomes progressively depressed. There are several reasons for this:
- Anaesthetic drugs build up progressively;
- The maternal placental circulation may be impaired by the supine position or by drugs;
- There may be progressive metabolic disturbance.

Whatever the cause of this progressive fetal depression, it is clear that a **short** procedure does not anaesthetise the baby. This is dependent on the techniques employed in this particular circumstance.

- First, no sedative or analgesic premedication is used for elective caesarean section.
- Secondly, a drug such as thiopentone which is used to induce anaesthesia is given by intravenous bolus (that is in a single shot) which maintains a concentration high enough to affect the maternal brain only for a short time, thereafter the concentration in the blood falls rapidly as the drug is dispersed to other sites in the mother. The same bolus of drug crosses the placenta as crosses the blood-brain barrier, but once across the placenta the drug undergoes further dilution in the baby's liver and blood stream. By the time it reaches the baby's brain it is too dilute to have a profound effect.
- Thirdly, drugs used to maintain anaesthesia build up slowly in the tissues of the mother and even more slowly in those of the baby.

4.3.3 Analgesia in labour

Although an analgesic such as pethidine produces negligible pain relief when given systemically in labour, it has been widely used and extensively studied. Fetal effects, such as reductions in fetal heart rate variability,[39] movement, breathing,[40] EEG activity and oxygen tension[41] have been discerned within minutes of administration to the mother. We know, however, that a single intramuscular dose of pethidine has negligible effect on the newborn if given to the mother within one hour of delivery, while maximal effects are seen when the dose delivery interval is more than 3 hours.[42,43] This is because, although pethidine crosses the placenta easily, it builds up slowly in the fetus, and more importantly, its primary metabolite, nor-pethidine, is a major cause of neonatal depression and accumulates even more slowly in the baby. It has long been recognised that maternal sedation throughout labour results in a very drowsy newborn.[44]

An intravenous injection of opioids such as fentanyl and alfentanil, and benzodiazepines such as diazepam, may have a depressant effect of more rapid onset than that of an intramuscular dose of pethidine. Though the effect may be observed in a few minutes in the fetus, it will be neither as quick nor as profound as that in the mother.

Most of our understanding of placental transfer of anaesthetic and analgesic drugs relates to late gestation, when the efficiency of the placenta as an organ of passive diffusion is at its maximum. Transfer of such substances earlier in pregnancy would be, if anything, only slower.

4.3.4 Chronic maternal drug administration

Lipid-soluble drugs given over a longer period than is required for anaesthesia or analgesia in labour can be expected to affect the baby in the same way as the mother, a placental barrier operating only for lipid-insoluble substances. Effective maternal sedation and analgesia over some hours can therefore confidently be expected to provide similar fetal effects.

4.3.5   *Effects on the stress response*

Maternal stress, such as that provoked by prolonged labour or any painful procedure, tends to have adverse effects on the wellbeing of the fetus; hence reassurance and effective pain relief for the mother are beneficial.[45] By contrast fetal stress plays an important positive role in adaptation to extrauterine life.[46] The stress response observed in babies following labour and vaginal delivery is substantially more marked than that following elective caesarean section. The stress response is suppressed in the baby by general anaesthesia, while it is preserved if epidural anaesthesia is used, and the effect of spinal anaesthesia is intermediate.[46] Cardiac function in the newborn is also impaired by general but not by regional anaesthesia,[47] an effect which presumably begins *in utero*.

Enthusiasm for administering powerful opioid analgesics to fetuses requiring invasive interventions needs to be tempered by the possibility that such administrations might cause long-term harm. Because the fetal nervous system undergoes dramatic maturational changes, including alterations in neurotransmitter receptor numbers and function, it is possible that opioid exposure at a critical stage of neural plasticity might alter the normal course of receptor development. These aspects deserve urgent research.[3] No such reservations should apply, however, to the mature fetus in a pregnancy that is about to be terminated.

5. Is there a need for change?

5.1 Use of analgesia

5.1.1 In continuing pregnancies

The available anatomical and physiological evidence informs us that thalamocortical connections do not penetrate the cortical plate before 26 weeks. Therefore although the fetus may show reactions, it cannot be aware of sensory stimuli before that time. After that time, the fetus will not instantly be able to feel pain. Cortical connections develop over a prolonged period. The developing cortex only gradually acquires the functional capacity to perceive sensory stimuli, to become aware of pain and eventually to remember the experience and to prompt a change in behaviour.

The Working Party concludes that it is not possible for the fetus to be aware of events before 26 weeks' gestation. Because of the uncertainty that attends estimates of gestational age, it may be appropriate to consider providing some form of fetal analgesia or sedation for major intrauterine procedures performed at or after 24 weeks' gestation in order to remove the possibility of **any** sensory information reaching the cortex.

However, having in mind the subsequent development of the fetal nervous system it is still debatable whether fetal analgesia or sedation should be given for intrauterine procedures. We remain largely ignorant of the effect of drugs on the developing brain. The Working Party is, therefore, not recommending any changes in current practice at the present time.

In every case where there may be a need to administer sedative, analgesic or anaesthetic drugs in connection with performing intrauterine procedures, each practitioner should balance the possibility of the fetus feeling pain and the adverse effects of noxious stimulation against the potential harm that may arise from the use of these drugs.

5.1.2 In termination of pregnancy

For terminations of pregnancy performed at 24 weeks or later, depending on the surgical procedure used, we recommend that:

EITHER, feticide should be carried out using a technique that stops the fetal heart rapidly such as injection of potassium chloride;[7]

OR, opioid or benzodiazepine premedication should be given to the mother and allowed sufficient time to cross the placenta and build up in the fetus (at least one hour for an intra muscular injection of pethidine for example, or 10-20 minutes for an intravenous injection) so as to sedate the fetus.

5.2 New research

The Working Party believes that further research should be undertaken in the following areas and that funding should be made available for this by appropriate bodies-

- The development of pathways for the transmission of noxious stimuli in the fetus and neonate.

- Placental transfer of analgesic drugs in the second trimester.

- The effect of analgesic drugs on stress responses in animal and human fetuses.

- Potential long term effects of intrauterine procedures, with or without analgesia.

- Animal research on the effects of opioids on the development of the fetal brain.

References

1. Hepper PG. Fetal memory: Does it exist? What does it do? *Acta Paediatrics* 1996;Supplement 416:16-20.

2. Kandel ER, Schwartz JH, Jessell TM. Cognition and the cortex. In: *Essentials of Neurological Science and Behaviour*. Connecticut: Appleton & Lange, 1995;347-363.

3. Aynsley-Green A. Pain and stress in infancy and childhood: where to now? *Journal of Paediatric Anaesthesia* 1996;**6**:167-172.

4. Jacobson, M. *Developmental Neurobiology*. New York: Plenum Press, 1991.

5. Taddio A, Goldbach M, Ipp M, Stevens B, Koren G. Effect of neonatal circumcision on pain responses during vaccination in boys. *Lancet* 1995;**345**:291-292.

6. Rice HE, Harrison MR. Open fetal surgery. In: Fisk NM, Moise KJ, eds. *Fetal Therapy: Invasive and Transplacental*. Cambridge: Cambridge University Press, 1997;27-35.

7. *Report of working party on termination of pregnancy for fetal abnormality*. Royal College of Obstetricians and Gynaecologists, London, 1996;15 and 21(Abstract).

8. Wall PD, Melzack R. *The Textbook of Pain*. London: Churchill Livingstone, 1994.

9. Fitzgerald M. Neonatal pharmacology of pain. In: Besson JM, Dickenson AH, eds. *Handbook of Experimental Pharmacology*, 1997.

10. Fitzgerald M. Pain in infancy: some unanswered questions. *Pain Reviews* 1995;**2**:77-91.

11. Fitzgerald M. The neurobiology of fetal pain. In: Wall PD, ed. *The Textbook of Pain*. London: Churchill Livingstone, 1994;153

12. Fitzgerald M. The development of pain pathways. In: Gluckman PD, Heymann MA, eds. *Perinatal and Paediatric Pathophysiology*. Edward Arnold, 1993;222-225.

13. Lloyd-Thomas AR, Fitzgerald M. Does the fetus feel pain? *British Medical Journal* 1996;**313**:795-796.

14. Humphrey T. Function of the nervous system in prenatal life. In: Stave U, ed. *Perinatal Physiology*. New York: Plenum Press, 1978;651-683.

15. Payne J, Middleton J, Fitzgerald M. The pattern and timing of cutaneous hair follicle innervation in the rat pup and human fetus. *Brain Research*; Developmental Brain:1991; 173-182.

16. Konstantinidou AD, Silos-Santiago I, Flaris N, Snider WD. Development of the primary afferent projection in human spinal cord. *Journal of Comparative Neurology* 1995;**354**:11-12.

17. Prechtl HF. Ultrasound studies of human fetal behaviour. *Early Human Development* 1985;**12**:91-98.

18. Hooker D. *The prenatal origin of behaviour*. Kansas: University of Kansas Press, 1952;

19. Andrews K, Fitzgerald M. The cutaneous withdrawal reflex in human neonates: sensitization, receptive fields, and the effects of contralateral stimulation. *Pain* 1994;**56**:95-101.

20. Casey KL, Minoshima S, Berger KL, Koeppe RA, Morrow TJ, Frey KA. Positron emission tomographic analysis of cerebral structures activated specifically by repetitive noxious heat stimuli. *Journal of Neurophysiology* 1994;**71**:802-807.

21. Mojsilovic J, Zecevic N. Early development of the human thalamus: Golgi and Nissl study. *Early Human Development* 1991;**27**:119-144.

22. Hasegawa M, Houdou S, Mito T, Takashima S, Asanuma K, Ohno T. Development of myelination in the human fetal and infant cerebrum: a myelin basic protein immunohistochemical study. *Brain & Development* 1992;**14**:1-6.

23. Khan AA, Wadhwa S, Bijlani V. Development of human lateral geniculate nucleus: an electron microscopic study. *International Journal of Developmental Neuroscience* 1994;**12**:661-672.

24. Sherman SM, Guillery RW. Functional organization of thalamocortical relays. [Review] [310 refs]. *Journal of Neurophysiology* 1996;**76**:1367-1395.

25. Klimach VJ, Cooke RW. Maturation of the neonatal somatosensory evoked response in preterm infants. *Developmental Medicine & Child Neurology* 1988;**30**:208-214.

25a. Zecevic N, Verney C. Development of catecholamine neurons in human embryos with special emphasis on the innervation of the cerebral cortex. *J. Comp. Neurol.* 1995; 351: 509-535

26. Mrzljak L, Uylings HB, Kostovic I, van Eden CG. Prenatal development of neurons in the human prefrontal cortex. II. A quantitative Golgi study. *Journal of Comparative Neurology* 1992;**316**:485-496.

27. Casey KL. *Pain and central nervous disease: the central pain syndromes*. New York: Raven Press, 1991.

28. Anand KJS, Hickey PR. Pain and its effects in the human neonate and fetus. *New England Journal of Medicine* 1987;**317**:1321-1329.

29. Aynsley-Green A, Ward Platt MP. Pain in infancy and childhood. In: David TJ, ed. *Recent Advances in Paediatrics*. Edinburgh: Churchill Livingstone, 1993;228-241.

30. Anand KJS, Sippell WG, Schofield NM, Aynsley-Green A. Does halothane anaesthesia decrease the metabolic and endocrine stress responses of newborn infants undergoing operations? *British Medical Journal* 1988;**296**:668-672.

31. Anand KJS, Sippell WG, Aynsley-Green A. Randomised trial of fentanyl anaesthesia in preterm neonates undergoing surgery:effects of the stress response. *Lancet* 1987;**1**:62-66.

32. Giannakoulopoulos X, Sepulveda W, Kourtis P, Glover V, Fisk NM. Fetal plasma cortisol and β-endorphin response to intrauterine needling. *Lancet* 1994;**344**:77-81.

33. Schulze S, Roikjaer O, Hasselstrom L, Jensen NH, Kehlet H. Epidural bupivacaine and morphine plus systemic indomethacin eliminates pain but not systemic response and convalescence after cholecystectomy. *Surgery* 1988;**103**:321-327.

34. Desphande S, Ward Platt MP, Aynsley-Green A. Patterns of the metabolic and endocrine stress response to surgery and medical illness in infancy and childhood. *Critical Care Medicine* 1991;**21**:S359-361.

35. Matthews DSF, Aynsley-Green A, Matthews JNS, Bullock RE, Cooper BG, Eyre JA. The effect of severe head injury on whole body energy expenditure and its possible hormonal mediators in children. *Paediatric Research* 1995;**37**:409-417.

36. Ward Platt MP, Tarbit MJ, Aynsley-Green A. The effects of anesthesia and surgery on metabolic homeostasis in infancy and childhood. *Journal of Paediatric Surgery* 1990;**25**:472-478.

37. Rolf AR. Treat the babies, not their stress responses. *Lancet* 1993;**342**:319-320.

38. Reynolds F. Placental transfer of drugs. *Current Anaesthesia and Critical Care* 1991;**2**:108-116.

39. Kariniemi V, Ammala P. Effects of intramuscular pethidine on fetal heart rate variability during labour. *British Journal of Obstetrics & Gynaecology* 1981;**88**:718-720.

40. Zimmer EZ, Divon MY, Vadasz A. Influence of meperidine on fetal movements and heart rate beat-to-beat variability in the active phase of labor. *American Journal of Perinatology* 1988;**5**:197-200.

41. Rosen MG, Scibetta JJ, Hochberg CJ. Human fetal electroencephalogram. III. Pattern changes in presence of fetal heart rate alterations and after use of maternal medications. *Obstetrics & Gynecology* 1970;**36**:132-140.

42. Kuhnert BR, Kuhnert PM, Tu A-SL, Lin DCK. Meperidine and normeperidine levels following meperidine administration during labor. II. Fetus and neonate. *American Journal of Obstetrics & Gynecology* 1979;**133**:909-914.

43. Morrison JC, Whybrew WD, Rosser SI, Bucovaz ET, Wiser WL, Fish SA. Metabolites of meperidine in the fetal and maternal serum. *American Journal of Obstetrics & Gynecology* 1976;**126**:997-1002.

44. Brackbill Y, Kane J, Manniello RL, Abramson D. Obstetric premedication and infant outcome. *American Journal of Obstetrics & Gynecology* 1974;**118**:377-384.

45.   Moore J. The effects of analgesia and anaesthesia on the maternal stress response. In: Reynolds F, ed. *Effects on the baby of maternal analgesia and anaesthesia.* London: Saunders, 1993;148-162.

46.   Irestedt L. The effects of analgesia and anaesthesia on fetal and neonatal stress responses. In: Reynolds F, ed. *Effects on the baby of maternal analgesia and anaesthesia.* London: Saunders, 1993;163-168.

47.   Hagnevik K, Irestedt L, Lundell B, Skoldefors E. Cardiac function and sympathoadrenal activity in the newborn after cesarean section under spinal and epidural anesthesia. *Acta Anaesthesiologica Scandinavica* 1988;**32**:234-238.